Hand Sanitizer Recipes:

Your Easy and Practical DIY Anti-Germ and Antivirus Guide for a Healthier and Safer Lifestyle

Paul S. Leland

Table of Contents

As a way of saying thanks for purchasing this book, there is a gift for you: a theme as topical as ever. Discover the dynamics of this sneaky invisible enemy to better protect you and your family.

Simply copy and paste the link below into your browser, to get your gift:

https://dl.bookfunnel.com/spqs3v2rnp

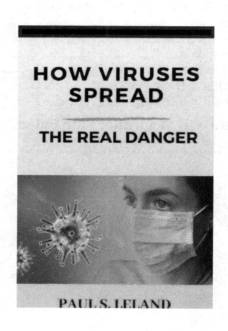

Introduction

Personal hygiene and, in particular, one of its fundamental rules that wash and disinfect your hands regularly, has never been as topical as it is now.

With the spread of diseases belonging to the coronavirus family, such as COVID-19, it is essential to understand why it is important to have hands to prevent the spread of potentially deadly germs.

Ask yourself these questions:

Do you prepare or eat your food and drink without washing your hands?

Do you touch surfaces or objects that are "at-risk", i.e., potentially "contaminated"?

Are you in the habit of touching your face with unwashed hands?

These are points to think about to improve your hygiene and avoid contracting viruses or bacterial infections of various kinds.

In the following chapters, we'll see how to use a hand sanitizer, which is the best technique to disinfect your hands, obtaining the best results to eliminate all the germs present.

We will also know the differences between alcohol-based and non-alcoholic disinfectants, what are their advantages and disadvantages.

We will see the steps to prepare a disinfectant and the materials you need, from the choice of gel or spray to the type of suitable container are. We will then follow a list of recipes to create disinfectants with pleasant fragrances, and this is the "operational" part, the most enjoyable and fun. You can have fun choosing and playing with the scents that best suit you.

In the end, you will also find a section dedicated to creating perfumed disinfectant wipes for you and your children.

In the first chapters, we talk about how you can stay safe using

homemade disinfectants. In this regard, essential oils play a crucial role, as potent plant extracts are beneficial to prepare a hand disinfectant. They are very suitable for their cleansing and soothing properties of the skin, as well as perfuming the compound by removing the typical odor of alcohol.
Well, then we can start having fun.

Chapter 1: The Axe Health-Washed Hands

We all wash our hands several times a day. It´s a routine operation, and we´re used to it by now. We carelessly because it´s part of our morning routine, when we wake up before eating, and maybe before going to bed in the evening. But have we ever stopped to understand the science behind this, at first sight, very standard action?

I am referring to what allows us to free our hands from pathogens that cause viruses and bacteria. There are a whole series of factors that affect and are involved in this essential operation, which can preserve our health.

The effectiveness of hand washing depends on how we use it, how intensely we rub it, and above all, how we dry it. Each step of this process has its importance, aimed at eliminating pathogens that are dangerous to health.

The Journey of Germs

They are everywhere. They are billions and billions. They spread in different ways, by air, and by direct and indirect contact.
Bacteria and airborne germs spread through airborne droplets even several meters away from sneezing or coughing.
But you can also get infected by grabbing a standard shopping cart, perhaps used by someone before us who had not washed his hands, or simply shaking hands when we greet someone. That´s how germs spread. There can be countless situations in which you can get infected, including the most common ones are touching the handles in places and public transport, in stations and airports, and so on. Everywhere we go, we encounter surfaces where bacteria are present.

We can use simple precautions, such as disinfecting our hands when we are out and about and have touched something, not touching our eyes, nose, and mouth, and, above all, washing our hands often. If we are out and about and this is not possible, it helps to have a hand sanitizer with us to protect our health and that of our loved ones.

For a disinfectant to be effective against germs, it should contain at least 60% alcohol, better if 90%, to eliminate all types of bacteria and viruses. Depending on personal taste, it´s possible to create an aromatic or neutral one. But this aspect we´ll see below.

Useful Tips

The recent global health emergency requires us to observe some simple rules more than we did before. Just remember to do so to avoid unpleasant problems.

The recent COVID-19 emergency has brought more awareness about the need to wash our hands:

- When you touch any surface or object in a public place, it may have been touched by other people. For example, tables, door handles, gas pumps, shopping trolleys, or electronic screens, and many others.
- When you´re in the office, at work, or home, it´s advisable to disinfect the surfaces you need, and then wash your hands. Please do the same before eating or touching food to prepare or cook it.
- If you have had contact with one or more people, affecting what they may have touched, disinfect your hands. Do the same before cleaning and dressing a wound or cut.
- Sanitize your hands after using the toilet. It also applies to your pet´s food or feces.
- After taking the garbage to the dumpster, always clean

your hands thoroughly.

Think about how many surfaces you touch from the moment you leave the house until you reach your workplace. Once in that space, how many covers are then touched by others. A lot, I'm sure.

Remember: Germs are challenging to remove if you ignore them!

Chapter 2: Effective Ways to Wash Your Hands

You must be sure you are thoroughly cleaning your hands using proper technique.

Washing your hands well and effectively does not just mean opening the water and spraying soap on them. There is a technique to eliminate the pathogens present on the skin of our hands.
A good result is a combination of several factors, such as the time and effectiveness of rubbing, the product you use, drying. Following the correct method allows us to preserve our health, which is no small thing!

So let´s see what an effective method to wash your hands is.

- Saturate your hands thoroughly with hot or cold tap water. The temperature is indifferent, and there are no indications about the effectiveness of bacteria elimination.
  However, keep in mind that water that is too hot can irritate sensitive and thin skin, while water that is too cold can lead to cracking of the surface of the hands, especially if it is cold.
- Please turn off the water tap, take the soap, whether liquid, in a bar or gel, and start rubbing your hands aggressively until they form a gentle foam. Make sure it covers the whole hand, and pass it under the fingernails and between the fingers. The friction created helps to lift the grease, dirt, and microbes from the skin. You need to rub your hands for no less than twenty to thirty seconds. It is the time required to eliminate pathogens and get clean hands.
- Then reopen the tap and rinse your hands thoroughly with hot, cold, or warm water, depending on your

preference.

- Use a clean towel or paper towels, and rub your hands for at least twenty seconds, taking care to dry all parts. A wet side has a very high probability of attracting germs and viruses, much more than a dry hand.

Germs are bacteria, which are pathogens capable of causing even severe diseases in humans.

It is essential to use clean running water. If you use stagnant water, your hands may recontaminate. We recommend that you open the tap and let the water run for a few dozen seconds before starting to wash your hands.

Chapter 3: Benefits of Hand Sanitizers

The use of a hand disinfectant without water offers several advantages over the regular use of soap and water. Before starting to wash, make sure you have removed any organic matter that may be present on the skin, such as food residue, dirt, or debris of various kinds.

Benefits of Using a Waterless Hand Sanitizer

Portability: As you may already have noticed, soap and water are not always available when you need them, especially if you are out and about: on the road, in the office, or a public place. Make sure you always keep a bottle of disinfectant in your bag, pocket, or the glove compartment of your car, ready to extinguish any germs present for adequate and continuous protection.

The use of the disinfectant is quicker and less irritating to the skin than soap; it is also very effective in quickly killing microorganisms. The essential oils contained in disinfectants can even improve skin texture.

Chapter 4: When & How to Use a Hand Sanitizer

The Best Answer:Having a hand sanitizer is the easiest and correct choice if you do not have access to soap and water.

The alcohol base must be at least 60%, which is the minimum. The ideal would be 90% and even more. This concentration would guarantee the elimination of all viruses and bacteria.

To remove germs well, you need to be sure you have removed as much grease or visible dirt from the surface of your hands as possible.
If traces of grease or grease are present, as well as chemicals, metals, or pesticides, disinfectants may not be 100% effective.

The Proper Technique Used for the Application of Hand Sanitizer

To use the disinfectant gel, act as follows:

- Pour your favorite gel on one hand
- Rub both hands for about 20-30 seconds, taking care to clean the fingers and under the nails, where dirt can easily lurk.
- Rub until the hands dry

Quick Fixes for Hand Sanitizing

Peroxide: When you need a quick disinfectant, use 3% hydrogen peroxide. Pour it into a spray bottle, and use it directly or diluted with a little water. It works to break down and decompose bacteria.

White distilled vinegar: You might be surprised, but this excellent disinfectant can destroy many pathogens, including salmonella and E.coli. Add essential oil or use it directly from the bottle, which contains about 5% solution. Vinegar has an antibacterial agent that kills about 99% of germs. It is also non-polluting, edible and non-toxic. Besides, the smell of vinegar is dispersed within minutes. If desired, add about 20 drops of oil using a combination, such as thyme, tea tree, lemongrass, or patchouli.

Tea tree essential oil: Mix about four ounces of water with ten drops of tea tree oil in a spray bottle. If it´s too similar to a standard antiseptic, you can add a few drops of lavender extract, some lemon juice, or even both to provide more anti- viral and antibacterial benefits.

Combination of Aloe with Eucalyptus: Prepare a four-ounce spray bottle with an ounce of juice or aloe vera gel. The aloe juice is less viscous, and blends well with the solution. Fill the rest of the container with hot water and shake it to use immediately.

Other Hand Sanitizing Options: Quick & Easy

#1:Use a small bottle and pour some water, leaving some space on top to add the following ingredients:

- o Lavender essential oil (5-10 drops)
- o Palmarosa oil (3 drops)
- o Eucalyptus & lemon oil (5 drops of each)
- Shake the contents and use the sanitizer as needed.

#2:Use an oil containing vitamin E (0.25 tablespoon). Add some to soften your hands naturally. The oil also increases its durability as it is a natural preservative.

#3: Make a quick hand sanitizing gel using aloe vera gel (.33 cup) and 99% rubbing alcohol (.66 cup).

On average, you should consider washing and or sanitizing

your hands at least once each hour.

Consider this natural blend with proven antiviral and antibacterial properties. It has no alcohol or chemicals to harm your skin:

Prepare a spray bottle (four ounces).
Use sterilized/distilled water. Fill ¾ of the bottle.
Add the following:

- Aloe vera gel (1 tbsp.)
- Add Essential Oils: Add 10 drops each:
    - Cinnamon,
    - Clove
    - Rosemary
    - Eucalyptus
- Add lemon/orange/grapefruit essential oil (20 drops of either)

Securely close the top of the spray dispenser and mix thoroughly.
Spray two or three times on your hands. Rub the mixture until dry.
Use the spray as needed.

Chapter 5: Alcohol-Free Sanitizers Vs. Alcohol-Based Sanitizers

Disinfectants are useful against many pathogens, such as viruses and bacteria, which can weaken your health daily.
For maximum effectiveness, the Food and Drug Administration strongly suggests that alcohol should have a minimum concentration of 60 to 95%.

We can opt for two choices: alcohol-based hand disinfectants, or without. The pros and cons of each should be considered.

Alcohol-based products contain isopropanol, an effective antiseptic to kill bacteria. However, these are highly flammable and have potential toxicity risks, especially when ingested, for example, by children. Thus, you should always check the use of disinfectants in the presence of your young children.

The world's leading health organizations such as the WHO, FDA, and CDC recommend alcohol-based products.

Alcohol-Free Hand Sanitizers

In today's market, most alcohol-free products consist of a water-based foam containing benzalkonium chloride, which is the active ingredient providing the same level of protection - even after drying. If desired, it can be enriched with skin conditioners, such as green tea extract or vitamin E. It is non-toxic and non-flammable.

Disadvantages of Alcohol-Based Hand Sanitizers

Dry Skin & Risks of Infection

The prolonged use of alcohol-based disinfectants can destroy the skin's natural oils. It can cause painful symptoms:

- Gray, ashy skin color
- Redness
- Light to severe peeling or flaking
- Itching
- Fine lines/cracks
- Bleeding from deep cracks in the skin

These conditions can provide the perfect environment for infection to enter your body.

Fire Hazard Risk

Many of the hand disinfectants available on the market today contain a high volume of alcohol. Alcohol-based hand disinfectants are classified as "class I flammable liquid substances", which means that they have a flash point below 100° Fahrenheit.

OSHA provides these guidelines for storage and use:

- Storage in a safe and cool place
- Always keep all hand sanitizers away from any source of ignition, such as an electrical outlet or flame
- Remove spilled disinfectants immediately with water
- Watch children when using disinfectants, as they may swallow them, especially perfumed ones

Chapter 6: Tools & Materials for Correct Preparation

Step #1: Decide Whether You Want a Gel or Spray

Spray hand sanitizers can have alcohol as a basic ingredient or witch hazel. Both require a small spray bottle.

Alcohol was already used as a disinfectant in the year 1363. But it´s only since the eighties that it started to be commonly used as hand disinfectant.

Alcohols To Use:

- *80% + Ethanol Products:* Select 160 proof or higher drinkable grain alcohols (found at the liquor store).

   190 proof *Everclear*(92.4% ethanol) *See the recipe below.*

   190 proof *Golden Grain* (95% alcohol)

   192 proof *Spirytus Vodka* (96% alcohol).

If you use vodka in a spray, be sure to select a minimum of 140 proof vodka.

- *Recipe For Hand Sanitizer Using Everclear*

   Materials Needed:

   - Everclear (1 cup)
   - Aloe vera (.33 cup)
   - Coconut oil (2 tbsp.)
   - Essential oil (2-3 drops)
   - Optional: Hydrogen peroxide (amt. depends on supply)

Isopropyl Alcohol, also called rubbing alcohol, can be found in the community drug store. (Choose alcohols of 91 to 99%). Isopropyl alcohol, also called rubbing alcohol, is found in ordinary pharmacies. (Choose alcohol from 91 to 99%).

Preparation Steps:

Combine everything in the chosen container.

Here are some suggestions of places to look for alcohol:

- Your local grocery store
- A drugstore or pharmacies
- Your corner store
- Online places like Amazon
- Office supply stores, such as Staples
- Walmart
- Target
- Hardware stores

Choose A Waterless Hand Sanitizer:

Materials Needed:
- Thieves essential oil (10 drops)
- Castile liquid soap (.5 tsp.)
- Distilled water
- *Also Needed:* Foaming soap dispenser

Preparation Steps:

1. Fill the container with liquid soap and Thieves oil

2. Pour the water required for foaming. however, the product will not foam as freely as commercial blends.

3. Shake the contents slightly until a complete mixture is obtained, after which it is ready for use.

Choose a Container

Plastic containers vs. glass ones. Traditionally hand sanitizers on the market are available in plastic containers, but your ingredients may interact with plastic and have long-term adverse effects on your health.
The advantages of glass are that it is BPA and lead-free.

Use amber or blue bottles. Amber glass containers offer UV protection for your finished product.
The spray glass bottle must be made of FDA approved materials, which means you can safely use them for any compound.
Besides, many essential oils are available in amber-colored containers.

Before starting the process, remember to disinfect and sterilize all the instruments you will use to prepare your homemade disinfectants. You can do this with a pot of boiling water on the stove. Wash your hands and instruments with soap and water and immerse the tools in the water in the pan.

Step #3: Shop for Natural Ingredients

Aloe Vera Gel: Unlike other aloe vera gels, the gel we want to use is not sticky. It is the one certified at 99.75% purity, with ¼ of its content composed of natural ingredients.
Glycerin: An ingredient in many liquid soaps, vegetable glycerin helps stabilize the hand disinfectant and also keeps hands soft. You can buy glycerol jugs online.

Grape seed oil: Use it as a moisturizer and to help give freshness to your product.

Vitamin E Oil. Vitamin E Oil is a great discovery because it nourishes and moisturizes the skin. Choose an unscented vitamin E oil.

Witch Hazel: As a disinfectant, it is ideal because it is antiseptic, antibacterial, anti-inflammatory, astringent, antifungal and antimicrobial.

Colloidal / ionic silver contains antibacterial properties. Silver has been the antibiotic of choice for years, until proprietary drugs were available.
You can buy a bottle of colloidal silver and use it 100% in the spray bottle. If desired, add five drops of cloves and eucalyptus to the silver..

Savvy Horsewoman's Hand Sanitizer

Materials Needed:
- 91% Rubbing alcohol (.5 cup)
- 14% alcohol - Witch Hazel (.25 cup)
- Pure aloe vera gel (.25 cup)
- Vegetable glycerin (.125 cup)
- Optional: Tea tree oil /Peppermint (5 drops)

Preparation Steps:

1. Pour the ingredients into a food processor or blender and run for about a minute.
2. Pour the mixture into the chosen container.
3. Store the bottle in a cool, dark place.

Choose the Fragrance or Not

Make the product what you like every time you disinfect your hands.

Label Your Product

The last but no less important step, to create your own hand sanitizer, is to label it.
A disadvantage in making homemade hand sanitizers is that you can forget what´s in the bottle! That´s why it becomes essential to apply a label on the bottle.
With labelling you end the confusion. You can find the labels online

Resources to create your own unique fantasy labels. Here are some labels for your hand sanitizers:
Love essential oil labels: You can use these free printable labels for a variety of homemade products.

Uniclife essential oil labels. These labels are made of handmade paper, suitable for labelling a multitude of items. Keeping your essential oils organized has never been so easy and fun. They are easy to peel off when you need them.
Compared to simple paper labels, handmade paper labels allow your writing to stay longer and not fade easily.

Chapter 7: List & Mixtures - Popular Essential Oils

An article in the American Journal of Essential Oils and Natural Products said some essential oils could help fight flu viruses, although further research is needed.

Preparing a hand disinfectant is quite simple, and requires no specific knowledge. We can achieve excellent effectiveness using two parts 99% alcohol and one part aloe vera.

Here's the example:

- 99% rubbing alcohol (.66 cup)
- Aloe vera gel (.33 cup)
- Choice of essential oils (10 drops)
- Bottle with small pump

Always remember that alcohol must be over 60% to kill germs.

Preparation steps:

1. Mix the aloe well.
2. Add the chosen oil and stir.
3. Pour the disinfectant into a bottle, using a funnel.
4. Fix the lid, shake it and start to kill the germs.

Create your blend of "thief's oil":

- Thieves oil is a mixture of several essential oils, generally the following:
- Cinnamon: Obtained from the bark, leaves, or twigs of different species of cinnamon.
- Clove nail: Made with the undeveloped buds of the flowers found on the Eugenia caryophyllata species of

the clove tree.
- Eucalyptus: Obtained from the leaves of eucalyptus plants, originating in Australia.
- Lemon: Extracted from the peel of the lemon fruit, Citrus limon
- Rosemary: derived from the herb rosemary, Rosmarinus officinalis

Potential Benefits of Thieves Oil

- Boosts immune function and fights infection. Strengthens the immune system
- Has antimicrobial activity
- Fight against nasal and sinus congestion
- Promotes respiratory and cardiovascular health
- It´s an energizing or uplifting mood enhancer

#1 Thieves' Oil

Essential Oils Needed:

- Clove bud (40 drops)
- Rosemary (10 drops)
- Lemon (35 drops)
- Cinnamon bark (20 drops)
- Eucalyptus (15 drops)

Preparation Steps:

1. Shake each oil well first, then pour them into a dark glass bottle. What we get is a highly concentrated solution.
2. Always dilute correctly before using it.

You can also create the "thieves' oil" blend by adding or replacing other essential oils.
For example, you might want to replace several oils with citrus fruits such as lemon, orange or bergamot.
Alternatively, you can add them to the traditional herbal recipe, such as thyme.
It would help if you tried to achieve the right balance of aromas to suit your taste.

Keep in mind that adding too intense an aroma could overwhelm the weaker ones..

#2 Thieves' Oil Blend

It is an excellent compound. Doesn´t tend to dry right away, though.

Essential Oils Needed:
- Lemon (9 drops)
- Clove (10 drops)
- Cinnamon (5 drops)
- Rosemary (3 drops)
- Eucalyptus (4 drops)

This is to make a cup of Thieves oil.

Materials Needed:
- Pure witch hazel (.33 cup)
- 100% aloe vera gel (.66 cup)
- Thieves' blend - #2 above (15 drops) (*Or below essential oils*)
  - Rosemary (1 drop)
  - Eucalyptus (2 drops)
  - Clove (5 drops)
  - Cinnamon (3 drops)
  - Lemon (4 drops)
  - Vitamin E oil (1 capsule)

"Thieves" Hand Sanitizer - Kid-Friendly 10 Years & Older

Use the above recipe for the blend.

Materials Needed:
- 1-ounce spray bottle
- Alcohol @ 95% (4 tsp.)
- Aloe gel (1 tsp.)
- Castille soap - unscented (1 tsp.)
- Thieves essential oil blend (6 drops)

Preparation Steps:

1. Fill the spray bottle with each of the components (oil and alcohol).

2. Shake the bottle and let it rest for about two hours.

3. After this time, mix the aloe and soap.

4. Close the lid tightly and shake the mixture again until it is well blended.

5. Label the container for safety

6. When it is ready to use, spray a portion on your hands. Rub the liquid and wait for it to dry.

Youngster-Friendly "Thieves" Hand Sanitizer - Six Months & Up

Ingredients:

- 1-ounce bottle
- Aloe gel (1 tsp.)
- Alcohol @95% (4 tsp.)
- Unscented Castille soap (1 tsp.)

Essential Oils:

- Cinnamon leaf (5 drops)
- Sweet orange (3 drops)
- Pine (2 drops)

Preparation Steps:

1. Fill the spray bottle with oils and alcohol.
2. Shake the mixture and let it rest for about two hours.
3. Add aloe to the spray bottle and secure the top firmly.
4. Shake well and label the bottle with its contents.
5. Spray on hands, and rub the liquid carefully from fingertips to wrist. Let it dry.

Benefits of Specific Essential Oils

Some essential oils are said to have antiviral properties, as well as antibacterial and antifungal properties.

<u>Bergamot</u> contains antibacterial elements, which help skin conditions, including eczema. It is also useful as a stress reducer.

<u>Chamomile</u> helps to relax and, at the same time, improves mood.

<u>Cinnamon bark oil</u> is an astringent, antifungal, antibacterial and antimicrobial. According to The New York Times, researchers recommend its application for the hands.

<u>Clove</u> is useful as an antiviral, antiseptic, antibacterial, antibacterial, and antifungal oil.

<u>Eucalyptus oil</u> is an excellent option to use as an antibacterial, antifungal, antiviral, antiseptic, and antimicrobial.

<u>Incense</u> contains antimicrobial properties and is a delightful option as a disinfectant.

<u>Geranium oil</u> is excellent as an antibacterial, antifungal, antiviral, and antiseptic.

<u>Jasmine</u> excels with a delicious aroma, which helps in times of depression—recommended during childbirth.

<u>Lavender</u> is excellent for stress relief. It has a refreshing and aromatic smell. It´s also an antiseptic, antiviral, antibacterial, antifungal, and antimicrobial oil.

<u>Lemon</u> is used for mood enhancement, digestion, and headache relief. Lemon essential oil is also a classic antiviral that works as an antibacterial, antifungal, antimicrobial, and antiseptic.

<u>Peppermint</u> is used to aid digestion and as an energy

stimulator. It also has antimicrobial properties that make it an excellent oil that typically works as an antiseptic, antibacterial, and antiviral. It provides a feeling of freshness.

Thyme essential oil has antibacterial qualities, but should not be used by children, as it may cause skin sensitivity. It is excellent as a hand disinfectant. It can also help prevent infection from cuts and scratches.

Rose helps reduce anxiety and improves mood.

Rosemary has a woody aroma and is known as a mild painkiller. It is also useful as an antiseptic, antibacterial, antifungal, and antimicrobial.

Sandalwood is used to aid concentration and calm the nerves.

Sweet orange oil is an antiseptic and is excellent for the skin to help fight sepsis and fungal infections. Orange essential oil increases immunity and eliminates toxins.

Tea tree oil is an antifungal, antiseptic, antibacterial, antimicrobial, antiviral, and is much used for the preparation of hand disinfectants.

Ylang-Ylang helps in certain skin conditions, but also for nausea and headaches.

More Delightful Combinations

- 3 drops Cinnamon Bark, 4 drops Lemon, 3 drops Eucalyptus Radiata

- 5 drops Thieves, 5 drops Tea Tree

- 4 drops Spearmint, 3 drops Lavender, 3 drops Bergamot

- 5 drops Purification, 5 drops Lemon

Chapter 8: Recipes for Basic Hand Sanitizers

You will find different ways to prepare your basic disinfectants and various recipes suitable for children. Always pump enough disinfectant on your hands (three to four pumps), then rub your hands thoroughly and let them dry. You will eliminate microbes, and your hands will feel clean and soft after the gel has dried.

Basic Hand Sanitizer Recipes

Equipment Needed:

- 2-ounce pump bottles
- Funnel
- Small bowl

Note: Store-bought aloe vera will last longer.

Hand Sanitizer With 99% Isopropyl Alcohol

- Isopropyl alcohol 99% (.75 cup)
- Aloe vera gel (.25 cup)
- Glycerin (1 tsp.)
- Essential oil (10 drops)

Hand Sanitizer With 70% Isopropyl Alcohol

- Isopropyl alcohol 70% (.75 cup)
- Glycerin (1 tsp.)
- Aloe vera gel (1.5 tbsp.)
- Essential oil (10 drops)

Hand Sanitizer With Witch Hazel

- Aloe vera gel (.25 cup)
- Witch hazel (.75 cup)
- Essential oil (10 drops)

Alcohol-Free Hand Sanitizer Gel

- Pure aloe vera gel (1 cup)
- Witch hazel - add until the desired consistency is reached (1-2 tsp.)
- Tea tree oil (25 drops or ¼ tsp. or increased amounts of other essential oils as desired)

Mostly Alcohol-Free Hand Sanitizer Gel

- Pure aloe vera gel (2 cups)
- 90% SD40 alcohol - perfumer's alcohol if you can get it (2 tbsp.)
- Tea tree oil or increased amounts of other essential oils (2-3 tsp.)

Alcohol-Based Hand Sanitizer

- Pure aloe vera gel (.25 cup)
- Grain alcohol or vodka (.25 cup)
- Tea tree oil or increased amounts of other essential oils (13 drops or ⅛ tsp.)

Hand Sanitizer - Blend Safe for Kids

Equipment Needed: Plastic or glass containers
Materials Needed:
- Aloe vera gel (.25 cup)
- Coconut oil (1 tbsp. - melted)
- Witch hazel - use low alcohol content (1.5 tbsp.)
  Essential Oils:
    - Lavender (5 drops)
    - Geranium (5 drops)

Preparation Steps:
1. Whisk the melted coconut oil and aloe thoroughly. Cool it if necessary.
2. Mix the rest of the fixings and pour it into the container.

Disinfecting Citrus Mint Hand Sanitizer - for Kids 10 + years

Equipment Needed:
- Spray bottle (1 ounce)

Materials Needed:
- Organic aloe gel (1 tsp.)
- 95% alcohol (4 tsp.)
- Unscented Castille soap (1 tsp.)

   Essential Oils:
   - Peppermint (2 drops)
   - Rosemary (5 drops)
   - Lemon (3 drops)

Preparation Steps:
1. Fill the spray bottle with the oils and alcohol.
2. Lightly shake the contents and let it set on the countertop for 2-3 hours.
3. Measure and mix in the soap and aloe into the bottle and tightly close the top.
4. Shake the bottle to mix the sanitizerthoroughly.
5. Label the spray with its ingredients.
6. When ready to use it, shake it and spray it on your hands. Rub the sanitizer into your skin and wait for it to dry.

Little Tykes Hand Sanitizer - for Kids 2-6 years old

Equipment Needed: Spray bottle (One-ounce)
Materials Needed:
- 95% alcohol (4 tsp.)
- Aloe gel (1 tsp.)
- Castille soap - unscented (1 tsp.)
  Essential Oils:
- Tea tree (1 drop)
- Lavender (2 drops)

Preparation Steps:
1. Fill the spray bottle with essential oils and the alcohol.
2. Thoroughly shake the bottle to mix the fixings.
3. Wait for two to three hours, so that the mixture can blend with its components.
4. Shake the ingredients and pour in the soapthoroughly. Close the top securely. Shake the ingredients thoroughly again.
5. Label the bottle. It is an important step to ensure your sanitizer remains safe and its ingredients active.
6. To Use: Spray on your hands. Rub the sanitizer into your hands thoroughly, and let it dry.

More Special Essential Oil Sanitizer Gels

Aloe Vera Fast Gel

Materials Needed:

- Leaf of the aloe plant
- Optional: For Each ¼ cup of gel - Add Vitamin E (400 IU) or Powdered Vitamin C (500 mg)

Preparation Steps:

1. Start the trial, "Wash your hands." It would help if you started with clean tools and hands to make sure the gel does not contaminate.
2. Slice the outer leaves of a mature aloe plant that contains the fresh, healthy gel.
3. Make a clean cut near the base of the plant. One or two large leaves should provide 0.5 to a cup of gel.
4. Put the leaves in a cup and let the resin drain for about ten minutes. The resin can slightly irritate the skin because it contains latex, so you don't want it in the gel.
5. Use a vegetable peeler to expose the green part on one side of each leaf to expose the gel layer. 5. Remove the gel with a large spoon and throw away the green leaves.
6. Prepare the mixture and add the vitamins if desired. 6. Blend the gel in a blender. At this stage, it will look foamy.
7. Add the gel into a clean, sanitized glass jar. It will last one to two weeks.
8. Use it in your recipes or for minor burns, skin irritations, minor wounds or insect bites. You can also mix ¼ cup of melted coconut oil with ½ cup of aloe for a moisturizing massage lotion. You can also apply a spoonful of gel to the scalp to relieve dandruff, as it contains cleansing, anti-inflammatory, and moisturizing elements.

9. Note: If you are not sure if you are allergic to the gel, test a small area before applying it to your hands. Wait a day or so.

Vodka-Type Gel Hand Cleanser

Equipment Needed: 8 oz. wide mouth container with lid
Materials Needed:
- Aloe vera gel (3 oz.)
- 190-proof vodka (5 oz.)
  Essential Oils:
    o Clove bud (20 drops)
    o Lemon (17 drops)
    o Cinnamon leaf (10 drops)
    o Eucalyptus (8 drops)
    o Rosemary (5 drops)

Preparation Steps:
1. Mix each of the oils in the container and add the alcohol. Secure the top closed and shake to dissolve the oils.
2. Open the lid and add the aloe. Shake it thoroughly. Toss it in a blender and mix if it clumps.
3. If you need one for on-the-go, add the mixture to that container, and you are ready to go.
4. Add a small bit of the gel to your hands when it's needed.

Large-Size Sanitizer Gel

The CDC recommends using at least 60% alcohol for hand sanitizers.

Any homemade recipe should be 2/3 alcohol to 1/3 aloe, or 2:1.

The following recipe made with grain alcohol, makes a disinfectant with just over 60%. For a disinfectant with a higher percentage of alcohol, increase the alcohol, and decrease the amount of aloe vera.

Equipment Needed:
- Glass pump bottle (4 oz.)

Materials Needed:
- Lavender oil (20 drops)
- Lemongrass oil (12 drops)
- of Clove Bud (10 drops)
- of Tea Tree oil (50 drops)
- Aloe Vera gel (2 oz./12 tsp.)
- Grain/Isopropyl alcohol or rubbing alcohol (4 oz./24 tsp.) or you can use witch hazel
- Grapeseed oil (2 tsp.)

Preparation Steps:
1. Prepare a small bowl with vitamin E and essential oils.
2. Mix in the alcohol/witch hazel and swirl the oils again.
3. Mix it all and pour it into clean - small spray bottles. The colored ones are best to help prevent light from exposing the ingredients.
4. Always gently shake the mixture before using it. It's good to use for several months.

Cinnamon Sanitizer Gel

Equipment Needed:
- Recycled soap bottle

Materials Needed:
- Distilled or boiled & cooled water (100 ml./approx. 3.4 oz.)
- *Essential Oils Needed - 15 drops each*:
  - Cinnamon
  - Lemon
- Aloe vera (2 tbsp.)

Preparation Steps:
1. Wash and sterilize the bottle before you begin.
2. Combine each of the recipe parts in the bottle.
3. Shake the mixture and use the gel as needed.

Eucalyptus Scented Gel Sanitizer

Equipment Needed:
- Recycled liquid soap /hand sanitizer bottle

Materials Needed:
- 99% rubbing alcohol - isopropyl alcohol, ethanol - grain alcohol (.66 cup)
- Aloe vera gel (.33 cup)
- Eucalyptus essential oil (8010 drops)

Preparation Steps:

Pour each of the ingredients into the chosen container.

Lavender Aroma Gel Sanitizer

Equipment Needed:

Materials Needed:

- Pure aloe vera gel (1 cup)
- Lavender essential oil (12 drops)
- Witch hazel (1-2 tsp.)

Preparation Steps:

1. Measure each of the components in a mixing bowl. If the mixture is too thin, add one teaspoon of aloe and so on, up to the desired point. Mix thoroughly.
2. Pour the disinfectant into a small bottle. Make sure to use a container without BPA, which can be found at your local pharmacy.

Outside the refrigerator, the solution will last up to three weeks.

Lavender & Cloves Gel

Equipment Needed:
- Small mixing bowl
- Small container for the gel

Materials Needed:
- Aloe vera gel (8 oz./16 tbsp.)
  Oils Needed:
    - Tea tree (25-30 drops)
    - Lavender & Clove oil (9 drops of each)
- Optional: Witch hazel (1 tbsp.)

Preparation Steps:
1. Prepare the mixing dish with the lavender and clove oils.
2. Add in the tea tree oil, the aloe, and witch hazel (if using).
3. Thoroughly mix and add it to the desired container.
4. You can use it for up to one month if stored out of direct sunlight and cold space.

Lavender & Lemon Hand Sanitizer

Equipment Needed:
- Flip-top container (2 oz.)

Materials Needed:
- Vegetable glycerin (2 tsp.)
- Rubbing alcohol at least 70% (2 tbsp.)
- Aloe vera gel (1 tbsp.)
  Essential Oils Needed:
    - Lemon & lavender (3 drops of each)
    - Tea Tree (4 drops)

Preparation Steps:

1. Combine aloe vera, vegetable glycerin, and alcohol in a shallow mixing container.
2. Mix the components thoroughly and add the essential oils.
3. Mix and add the mixture into the container using a funnel.

Lemon + 4-Essential Oil Hand Sanitizer - Kid-Safe

Materials Needed:
- Lemon oil (20 drops)
- Filtered water (3 oz.)
- Aloe vera gel (1 tsp.)
- *Essential Oils Needed - 10 drops of each:*
  - Cinnamon
  - Clove
  - Rosemary
  - Eucalyptus

Preparation Steps:
1. Prepare a four-ounce spray dispenser and shake the container gently to mix.

You can spray this on children's hands also.
It's chemical-free and helps keep germs away.

Plant-Based Hand Sanitizer

Materials Needed:
- Spray bottle (4 oz.)
- Sterile water (3 oz.)
- Aloe vera gel (1 tbsp.)
- Essential oils (10 drops each):
  - Rosemary
  - Clove
  - Cinnamon
  - Eucalyptus
- Lemon or orange (20 drops)

Preparation Steps:
1. Fill the spray bottle with the water.
2. Add the aloe gel and the above essential oils.
3. Shake the mixture thoroughly.
4. Spray your hands two or three times, then rub in the sanitizer.
5. Use this application anytime.

The Better (Spray) Recipes

You can replace the aloe vera gel with other alcohol. If the skin is sensitive, this type of disinfectant can dry it out.

You can make an organic, non-toxic hand sanitizer with simple ingredients:

- Distilled water
- Vodka
- Water
- Vegetable glycerin and
- Essential oils
- Isopropyl alcohol
- Hydrogen peroxide
- Glycerol or glycerin
- Spray bottle

However, Who recommends the following recipe. It is more powerful and less sticky.

Materials Needed:
- Alcohol (12 fl. oz.)
- Glycerol (2 tsp.)
- Hydrogen peroxide (1 tbsp.)
- Distilled/boiled & cooled water (3 fl. oz.)

Preparation Steps:

1. Mix the alcohol with glycerol, then peroxide with water. Mix it all. Add a splash of essential oil if desired.
2. Pour the mixture into a spray bottle.

Note: If you cannot find glycerol, proceed anyway, but you will need to moisturize your hands after applying the disinfectant. If you make a solution with low alcohol concentration, compensate for using less water. You will need at least ¾ of your final mixture to be alcohol.

Kid-Friendly Hand Sanitizer Spray

Equipment Needed:
- 2-oz. glass spray bottle

Materials Needed:
- Vegetable glycerin (.5 tsp.)
- *Essential Oils*:
  - Tea tree (20 drops)
  - Spruce (10 drops)
  - Lemon (6 drops)
- 190 proof vodka (alcohol) or at least 120 proof alcohol or 70% or higher isopropyl rubbing alcohol (.75 tbsp.)

Note: The original recipe included witch hazel. However, the best alcohol is the one recommended here. Please, do not use other types of alcohol (methanol, butanol) because they are toxic.

Preparation steps:
1. Add the glycerin and essential oils to the spray bottle.
2. Add the alcohol until the bottle is almost full.
3. Close the container and shake it carefully to combine the ingredients.

Gently shake the bottle. Spray freely on hands and rub together until dry.

Note: The use of vegetable glycerine provides moisturizing benefits, as alcohol can be very dry. If you choose to skip the essential oils (that are not optional), you could use aloe vera.

Moisturizing Anti-Bacterial Hand Sanitizer Spray - Method 1

Materials Needed:
- Rubbing alcohol - at least 60% concentration (1 tsp.)
- Aloe vera gel - 100% pure (.25 cup)
- Tea tree & Cinnamon and essential oils (10 drops of each)
- Antibacterial essential oils - ex. lavender, vanilla, lemongrass, peppermint, and orange (20 drops total)
- Distilled water
- Optional: Vegetable glycerin (.5 tsp.)

Preparation Steps:

1. Mix the alcohol, aloe gel, and glycerin in a mixing container.
2. Add the essential oils and mix thoroughly.
3. Pour in the distilled water until the mixture reaches the desired consistency.

Use a small funnel or a medicinal dropper to add it to the smaller bottles.

Moisturizing Hand Cleanser Spray - Method 2

Equipment Needed:

- Glass spray bottle (2 oz.)

Materials Needed:

- Vegetable glycerine (.5 tsp.)
- Thieves essential oil blend (5 drops)
- Vitamin E (.25 tsp.)
- Tea tree essential oil (3 drops)
- Almond oil (.5 tsp.)
- Witch hazel (1 tbsp.)
- Distilled water (as needed)

Preparation Steps:

1. Add each of the ingredients into the bottle. Fill the bottle with water.
2. It can be used for up to six months.

Ultra Sanitizer Spray

Materials Needed:
- 96% Ethyl alcohol (833 ml.)
- 3% hydrogen peroxide (42 ml.)
- 98% glycerin (15 ml.)
- Boiled/distilled water (up to 1 liter)

Preparation Steps:

1. Sterilize a one-liter glass bottle, or other container with the sprayer.
2. Remove thedistilled water and pour all fixings into the bottle.
3. Attach the lid securely.
4. Wait 72 hours before using the sprayer.
5. After the waiting time, shake and spray as desired.

Vinegar Disinfectant Spray

Equipment Needed:
- Spray bottle (100 ml.)

Materials Needed:
- Apple cider/white vinegar (49 ml.)
- Boiled & cooled/distilled water (49 ml.)
- Antibacterial essential oils of choice (40 drops)

Preparation Steps:

1. Measure and add all of the ingredients in the spray bottle.
2. Close the cap and shake until the components are thoroughly combined.
3. Spray your hands with the solution when needed.
4. Vinegar won't irritate your skin, and it also has a high disinfectant power. It's more intense with hydrogen peroxide. This mixture is also excellent for cleaning and

Chapter 9: The Importance of a Hand Sanitizer for Your Health In Life

You might want to try new blends, maybe for the changing seasons. Your health may improve when you take those extra 20 seconds during the day to disinfect your hands.

Try This Natural-Based Hand Sanitizer Formula:
- Small squeeze bottle
- Aloe vera gel (4 oz.)
- Essential Oils:

  - Peppermint (12 drops)
  - Sweet orange (14 drops)
  - Tea tree (22 drops)

Preparation Steps:
1. Add the mixture to the bottle.
2. Shake it fully before using it.

Create unique blends

Goodbye Allergy Blend: a combination of lemon, lavender, and peppermint.
Happy Blend: Enjoy the delicious combination of vanilla, lemon, orange, bergamot, and grapefruit.
Focus Blend: The aromas provided by incense, cedarwood, sandalwood, and vetiver are unmistakable.
Deep Breath Blend: Eucalyptus, cardamom, peppermint, lemon, rosemary, and tea tree are excellent for breathing.
Immune Boosting Blend: These oils are invigorating aromas, including cinnamon leaf (the bark would be strong), cloves, eucalyptus, rosemary, orange, and lemon.
Sleepy Time Blend: These are delicious blends to use in a bath container, including Roman chamomile, lavender, and vetiver.

Christmas Blend: Prepare some of these unique blends, including fir (balsamic fir, Douglas fir, silver fir), peppermint, and vanilla.

Sanitizer 1: Soothing Time

Materials Needed:
- Water (3 tbsp.)
- *Essential Oils*:
    - Bark oil or cinnamon leaves (2 ml.)
    - Eucalyptus & lemon (4 ml. of each)

Preparation Steps:
1. Combine each of the components.
2. Since water and essential oils do not mix naturally, the disinfectant must be shaken before use.
3. Thyme and oregano oils are also a vital component in fighting bacteria.

Note: Some have reported that cinnamon oil can cause some skin irritation. If this occurs, add more water to the recipe or replace the cinnamon with tea tree oil.

Sanitizer 2: Kitchen Delight

Materials Needed:
- Alcohol (1 tbsp.)
- Aloe Vera juice (3 tbsp.)
- *Essential Oils*:
  - Cinnamon (2 ml.)
  - Tea tree (3 ml.)
  - Lemon or lemongrass (3 ml.)

Preparation Steps:
1. Mix each of the fixings.
2. Shake the contents before using it.

Sanitizer 3: Sanitizer Body & Surface

Materials Needed:
- Aloe Vera gel (3 tbsp.)
- *Essential Oils*:
    - Lemon (5 ml.)
    - Tea tree (4 ml.)
    - If Desired: Thyme (2 ml.)

Preparation Steps:
1. Add the ingredients into the bottle.
2. Shake the container used each time before using it.

Special note: it can also disinfect surfaces such as those of your furniture. Make sure to test a small area first.

Sanitizer 4: A Natural Emulsifier

Materials Needed:
- Aloe vera (.5 cup)
- Lecithin (.5 tsp.)
- *Essential Oils*:
  - Thyme (1 ml.)
  - Lithium (1 ml.)
  - Orange (2 ml.)

Preparation Steps:
1. Combine the lecithin (a natural emulsifier) with the essential oils.
2. Slowly pour the mixture into the aloe, stirring as you go.
3. Lecithin is easily spotted as a bright yellow ingredient and can typically be found in health food stores.

Sanitizer 5: Winterbloom Delight

Materials Needed:
- Winterbloom extract (100 ml.)
- Essential oils such as lemon balm, eucalyptus, orange, cloves, cinnamon, and rosemary (5 drops total)
- Lemon essential oil (10 drops);
- *Optional*: Vitamin E/liquid coconut oil (2 tsp.).

Preparation Steps:

1. Prepare the disinfectant in a glass bottle with a spray dispenser.
2. Pour the Winterbloom into the bottle and add coconut oil/vitamin E.
3. Shake well. Add the desired essential oils and shake again.

Sanitizer 6: Peaches - Cinnamon & Lavender

Materials Needed:
- Aloe gel (3 tbsp.)
- *Essential Oils Needed - 5 drops of each*:
  - Lavender
  - Cinnamon
- Peach seed oil (5 drops)
- Tea tree oil (10 drops)
- Vitamin E (5 drops)

Preparation Steps:
1. Mix the cinnamon and tea tree oil together with the aloe.
2. Stir in the peach seed oil and Vitamin E. Fold in the lavender and mix well.
3. Shake the container before using it each time.

Sanitizer 7: Peppermint Delight

Materials Needed:
- Vitamin E
- Alcohol tincture of yarrow and calendula
- Your choice of base oils: Peach, almond, apricot. or sesame
- Peppermint essential oil (5 drops)

Preparation Steps:
1. For a liquid mix, combine the alcohol tincture of herbs and the base oil (one or a mixture) in a ratio of 2: 1.
2. You should have a 1:1 ratio for the gel solution.
3. Mix in the peppermint oil and Vitamin E to the sanitizer mixture.
4. Shake the container thoroughly to use.

Sanitizer 8: Cinnamon & Clove Specialty

Materials Needed:
- Liquid coconut oil (5 ml.)
- Alcohol tincture or alcohol (20 ml.)
- Pure distilled water (100 ml.)
- Cinnamon essential oil & cloves (5 drops)

Preparation Steps:

1. Join the compounds carefully and pour it all into a spray bottle.

2. If you do not have coconut oil, you can use olive, almond or peach oil as a substitute.

   This recipe is rich in benefits:

a) It has a robust microbicidal action, completely destroying microorganisms.

b) The solution has a presence of active substances that do not aggravate the resistance of the microflora.

c) The mixture has a prolonged antimicrobial action.

Sanitizer 9: Simple & Superb

Materials Needed:
- Tea tree oil (10 drops)
- Vitamin E (1 scant teaspoon)
- Water (150 ml.)

Preparation Steps:
1. Prepare the mixture in the chosen container.
2. Store it in a dark place between uses.

Sanitizer 10: Grapefruit & Lavender Splash

Materials Needed:
- Aloe Vera gel (1 tsp.)
- Sterile water (100 ml.)
- Tea tree oil (5 drops)
- Grapefruit oil (10 drops)
- Lavender extract (5 drops)
- Broth of herbs (50 ml.) mix one tsp. of sage, wormwood, and thyme - mix with boiling water (150 ml.)

Preparation Steps:
1. Prepare the broth of herbs. Pour it in the boiling water. Prepare these in a 10-minute water bath.
2. Combine the aloe with the lavender and tea tree oil. Shake them and add the sterile water. Mix this with the broth of herbs.
3. Pour the mixture into a spray bottle.

Chapter 10: Easy Sanitizer Wipes Preparation

The World Health Organization says you need to clean the surfaces you come into contact with daily to avoid the spread of germs, but it is essential to wash your hands with soap and water or, failing that, use a hand sanitizer.

In times like the present, with fears of the CoViD-19 pandemic, wipes in most stores have been sold out - nationwide. If you can't find them, use some of these handy recipes to help clean your surfaces.
As you know, wipes purchased in stores are expensive, so why not make your own, since they are cheaper to use?

If you decide to use bleach, add two teaspoons of household bleach to two cups of water. Avoid mixing bleach with anything other than water.

Be sure to cover all of these surfaces.

The Kitchen
- Light switches
- Countertops
- Trash cans
- Refrigerator handles
- Cabinet & drawer pulls
- Faucet & spray handle
- Oven handle & knobs

The Bathroom

- Countertops
- Doorknobs
- Faucets
- Light switches

- Toilet

Around the Home

- Remote controls
- Computer mouse
- Phones
- Thermometers
- Light switches
- Doorknobs

Outside Your Home

- The steering wheel & gear shift in the car
- Restaurant table
- Airplane – all surfaces
- Shopping cart

Alcohol

It is ingredient No 1 for the preparation of a disinfectant wipe. Make the disinfectant wipes by taking a paper towel or handkerchief, dab in alcohol (or another type of solution that is at least 60 percent alcohol), and clean any surface you want to clean.

The Best Essential Oils Containing Disinfecting Properties

Tea tree (Melaleuca alternifolia) is the species of tall shrub/tree in the myrtle family.

Lavender (Lavandula) is a genus of flowering plants in the mint family.

Geranium (Pelargonium) is a genus of flowering plants of succulents, perennials, and shrubs.

Lemon (Citrus limon) is a species of small evergreen trees in the flowering plant family - Rutaceae.

Orange (Citrus sinensis) is a small tree in the citrus family that originated in China.

Eucalyptus (Eucalyptus globulus) is a species of tall, evergreen tree endemic to southeastern Australia, and is also known as southern blue gum.

Rosemary (Rosmarinus officinalis) The name "rosemary" derives from Latin ros marinus ("dew of the sea").

Cinnamon (Cinnamomumverum) is a spice obtained from the inner bark of several tree species.

Cloves (Syzygiumaromaticum) are the aromatic flower buds of a tree in the family Myrtaceae.

Thyme (Thymus vulgaris) belongs to the family of the genus Thymus of aromatic perennial evergreen herbs in the mint family.

Peppermint (Mentha × Piperita) is a hybrid mint, a cross between spearmint and watermint.

Bleach Without the Fumes

Materials Needed:
- Distilled water (1 cup)
- Liquid castile soap (1 tsp.)
- Baking soda (.5 cup)
- Tea tree oil (20-30 drops)

Preparation Steps:
1. Combine each of the fixings for a superb ultra-powerful bleach alternative.

#1 Homemade "Clorox" Wipes

Equipment Needed:
- Rags cut into squares - ex. old washcloths are an excellent option: 24 (4 by 6-inches)

Materials Needed:
- Water (1 cup)
- Rubbing alcohol (.25 cup)
- Dawn dish soap (1 tsp.)
- Optional: Ammonia (2 tbsp.)

Preparation Steps:
1. Combine each of the fixings. Pour the mixture over the prepared rags.
2. Be sure to close the container with the rags and liquids securely.
3. Clean the spaces just as you would a regular disposable wipe. If you are using cloth, wash them if desired, and reuse the batch of clean wipes.

#2 Version Clorox-Style Wipes

Equipment Needed:
- Glass jar with a sealing lid
- Washcloths (10)

Materials Needed:
- Rubbing alcohol (2 cups)
- Dawn dishwashing soap (2-3 tsp.)
- Lemon essential oil (10 drops)

Preparation Steps:
1. Either leave the washrags whole or cut them into halves for smaller jobs.
2. Fill the chosen container with the rags.
3. Mix the alcohol, oil, and Dawn in a mixing dish.
4. Pour the cleaning mixture into the jar over the washcloths.
5. Place the lid on the container and use them when needed.
6. These are an economical option. Add the dirty rags to a jar to wash for the next time you prepare a new batch of the cleaner.
7. Note: Wipe the non-porous surfaces and let them dry (about ten minutes.)

#3 Quick Version Bleach Wipes - CDC Guided

Equipment Needed:
- Sturdy paper towels (1 roll)
- Sharp knife
- Airtight container (2)

Materials Needed:
- Water (2 cups)
- Bleach (1 tbsp.)

Preparation Steps:
1. Use a knife to saw/cut the roll of towels in half.
2. Mix the water and bleach in a mixing cup.
3. Remove the cardboard centers.
4. Put both halves of the roll of towels in one or two containers.
5. Pour the bleach solution over the rolls and close the lid.
6. Use them onsurfaces as needed.

Bathroom & Kitchen Cleaning Wipes

Equipment Needed:
Materials Needed:

- Distilled water (.75 cup)
- White vinegar (.25 cup)
- Unscented Castile liquid soap (.5 tsp.)
- *Essential oils - 10 drops each:*
    - Lemon (Citrus limon)
    - Tea tree (Melaleuca alternifolia)
    - Eucalyptus (Eucalyptus Radiata)

Preparation Steps:

1. Measure and add the water to a glass canister. You can substitute boiled and cooled filtered water for the distilled water

2. Add the vinegar and soap with 30 essential oil drops.
3. Gently stir the ingredients. Do not stir briskly, since it will cause the castile soap to bubble too much.
4. Prepare the guest towels or paper towels (your preference). Be sure the product is high-quality that will sustain the cleaning chores you have designated. Cut them in half and roll them into the jar, so they are in a ‚swirl.‘ This makes the removal of the towels much easier.
5. Securely close the lid and let the liquid work its way up the towels.

Economical Canister of Cleaning Wipes

Equipment Needed:
- Paper towel roll
- One-Pound coffee canister with a plastic lid
- Sharp knife
- Craft needle
- Scissors
- Optional: Spray paint

Materials Needed:
- Vinegar (.5 cup)
- Water (.25 cup)
- Rubbing alcohol (.25 cup)
- Liquid dish soap (1 tsp.)
- Optional: Essential oil (10 drops)

Preparation Steps:
1. Combine the water, alcohol, soap, and vinegar in a mixing bowl. Add the essential oil of choice to personalize its aroma for the space intended. You have several types to choose from to boost the antibacterial elements in the wipes.
2. Slowly add the liquid over the towels. After they are saturated, simply pull the towel cardboard from the center to create a feed for the wipes.
3. Use a large craft needle to pierce the middle of the lid. Push the scissors through the holes to create an opening of about ½-inch in diameter.
4. Feed the towel through the lid, and you are ready to disinfect your home's surfaces.

Reusable Disinfecting Wipes

Equipment Needed:
- Flannel baby wipes - 1- or 2-ply (8ǀ x 8ǀ size)
- 1 baby wipe container

Materials Needed:
- Warm filtered or distilled water (1 cup)
- Liquid Castile soap (ex. - Dr. Bronner's (1 tbsp.)
- Rubbing alcohol (.5 cup)

  Optional Essential Oils - 5 drops of each:
  - Tea tree
  - Lavender

Preparation Steps:
1. Combine the water, alcohol, soap, and vinegar in a mixing bowl. Add the essential oil of choice to personalize its aroma for the space intended. YOu have several types to choose from to boost the antibacterial elements in the wipes.
2. Slowly add the liquid over the towels. After they are saturated, simply pull the towel cardboard from the center to create a feed for the wipes.
3. Use a large craft needle to pierce the middle of the lid. Push the scissors through the holes to create an opening of about ½-inch in diameter.
4. Feed the towel through the lid, and you are ready to disinfect your home's surfaces.

Organic Hand Sanitizer Travel Wipes

Equipment Needed:
- Paper towels (1 roll)
- Storage container with a lid

Materials Needed:
- Coconut oil (1 tbsp.)
- Hot water (1.5 cups)
- Rubbing alcohol or vodka - ethyl alcohol (1 tsp.)
- Lemon and lavender essential oils (3 drops each)

Preparation Steps:
1. Mix the oils, water, and alcohol in a convenient travel-sized container. Wait for the coconut oil to melt into the liquid completely.
2. Remove the cardboard center of the paper towel roll and cut it into half. Place the towels in the container.
3. Add plenty of the mixture over the towels to wet them. Wait for them to soak in the liquid. Close the lid of the container.
4. Tip: For a sturdier wipe, don't use regular paper towels; choose using baby wipes or napkins.

#1 DIY Disinfectant Wipes

Equipment Needed:
- Tupperware container

Materials Needed:
- Warm water (2 cups)
- Rubbing alcohol - 70% alcohol minimum (1 cup)
- Dish soap (1 tbsp.)

Preparation Steps:
1. Combine everything and shake or stir it until blended.
2. Add the mixture to half a roll of paper towels in a Tupperware container.
3. Close the lid.

#2 Disinfecting Wipes

Materials Needed:
- Alcohol - isopropyl alcohol/rubbing alcohol or grain alcohol with a minimum of 140 proof (3 cups)
- 3% hydrogen peroxide (.75 tsp.
  Essential Oils Needed:
  - Lemon (20 drops)
  - Clove (15 drops)
  - Cinnamon bark (10 drops)
  - Eucalyptus Radiata oil & rosemary (5 drops of each)

Preparation Steps:
1. Pour about two cups of alcohol and hydrogen into the container.
2. Add the oils and mix well.

Prepare the Disinfectant Towels:
1. Always be sure to choose a high-quality (thick) paper. The paper needs to be tough enough to withstand the product and cleaning process.
2. You should prepare about thirty to forty dinner napkins or paper towels.
3. Fold each of the paper towels in half and stack them layered on top of each other.
4. Swirl the liquids around, leaving some in the bottom to help keep the towels moistened.

#3 Disinfecting Wipes

Equipment Needed:
- Old rags or paper towels

Materials Needed:
- Grain alcohol - 190 proof (1 cup)
- Distilled water (.25 cup)
- White vinegar (2 tbsp.)
- Dishwashing liquid soap (1 tsp.)
- Optional: Your choice - essential oils (8-10 drops)

Preparation Steps:
1. Combine each of the components in a mixing container.
2. If you use paper towels, cut the roll in half and tear off half sheets, so when you pull one, the next one will fold. Fold 25 towels in each stack.
3. Place the stacks into quart-size zipper baggies.
4. Pour in half of the mixture (on all sides of the bag for even soaking).
5. Seal the bag until it is needed. Slice a hole in the top and use it on the countertop as needed.
6. When it's not in use, cover it with tape or place it in another bag for another day.

Tips for Using Disinfectant Wipes:

1. Select a container with an airtight lid so that it can be shaken occasionally to distribute the liquids.

2. Make sure the container is made from materials safe to use with the diluted essential oils. Stainless steel, glass, and certain types of plastic (plastic #1 HDPE or plastic #2 PET) work for the job.

3. The chosen container needs to be large enough to hold the three cups of disinfecting solution plus thirty to forty paper towels.

To Use The Wipes:
1. Preclean any surfaces using an all-purpose cleaner before wiping it with the disinfectant wipes.
2. Pull a sanitizing wipe from the holder, making sure that the wipe is fully saturated with the sanitizing solution.
3. Wipe all hard surfaces with the sanitizing wipe until the surface is wet.
4. Leave the disinfected surface wet for about four to five minutes or wait for it to dry.

Disinfectant Spray for Surfaces

Materials Needed:
- High proof alcohol
- Hydrogen peroxide (.5 tsp.)
- Essential oils
- Spray bottle

Preparation Steps:
1. Apply this spray to highly-used areas like doorknobs, countertops, light switches, toilets, and sinks to help ward off sickness.
2. In addition to sanitizing, the spray can also be used to deodorize stinky surfaces like trash cans, furniture, shoes, and athletic equipment, and it can prevent mildew as well.

Chapter 11: Homemade Baby Wipes

#1 Baby Wipes

Equipment Needed:
- Airtight jar/container
- Paper towel roll (half of 1)

Materials Needed:
- Coconut oil (2 tbsp.)
- Baby wash - unscented (2 tbsp.)
- Filtered water (2 cups)
- Tea tree essential oil (3 drops)

Preparation Steps:
1. Use a microwavable measuring cup to heat the water for 1.5 minutes.
2. Scoop the oil and baby wash, and essential oil to the mix. Whisk them thoroughly until it's dissolved.
3. Cut a towel roll in half using a serrated knife. Put the towel into the jar.
4. Pour the mixture over half of the towel roll and wait for about one to two minutes.
5. After they are fully saturated, remove the cardboard tube. You can now easily pull the wipes from the center of the tube.
6. Place the lid tightly on the container and use as needed.

#2 Baby Wipes

This method will provide you with a box of wipes for less than one dollar! You can also add your option of essential oils for more bacterial protection.

Equipment Needed:
- Bounty paper towels/other similar option (1 roll)
- Square or round container (7-8 cup capacity)

Materials Needed:
- Water (2 cups)
- Liquid baby bath soap (2 tbsp.)
- Baby oil (1 tbsp.)

Preparation Steps:
1. Cut the paper towel roll in half with a serrated or bread knife.
2. Place one of the halves in the chosen container. Set the second half in the pantry until you are ready to make another batch.
3. Boil the water for two minutes.
4. Pour the liquid bath soap and baby oil into the boiled water.
5. Pour mixture evenly over paper towels.
6. Pull out the cardboard core of the paper towel roll. It comes out easily once it is wet.
7. Place the lid on the container.
8. Keep the lid securely on the container until ready to use.
9. Start by pulling the wipes from the center of the roll, and then replace the lid after each use.
10. The wipes should stay wet and fresh for up to a week. If you haven't used all of the wipes and they start to dry out, add some boiled water to refresh the roll.
11. Never flush the wipes!

#3 Natural Baby Wipes

Equipment Needed:
- Heavy-duty paper towels (1 roll like Bounty)
- Rubbermaid #6 or #8 container

Materials Needed:
- Pure witch hazel extract (1 tbsp.)
- Distilled/boiled water (1.75 cups)
- Pure aloe vera (1 tbsp.)
- Liquid castile soap - ex. - Dr. Bronner's (1 tsp.)
- *Optional:*
    - Grapefruit Seed Extract (10 drops) or Vitamin E (2 capsules)
    - Olive/almond oil (1 tsp.)
    - Essential oils of choice (ex. 6 drops each of orange and lavender)

Preparation Steps:
1. Use a sharp knife to sever the roll of towels into halves.
2. Place the wipes, cut side down in the chosen container.
3. Use a quart-sized jar or mixing container to combine the components. Stir well and pour the mixture over the towels in the jar.
4. Flip the jar over to soak each of the towels.
5. If your baby has sensitive skin, you may want to omit the essential oils or use a chamomile or calendula oil.
6. Note: For the containers, you can also use old wipes containers, old plastic coffee containers, plastic shoe box containers, or empty gallon plastic ice cream buckets.

#4 Budget-Style Baby Wipes

Materials Needed:
- Bounty paper towel roll (half of 1) $.37
- Organic virgin coconut oil (1 oz.) $.59
- Dr. Bronner's Soap (1 oz.) $.40
- Water (2 cups) free

Preparation Steps:
1. Boil the water to help prevent mold.
2. Cut the paper towel roll in half.
3. Combine each of the ingredients. The coconut oil will also help prevent mold. The oil should be about 76° Fahrenheit, so that it will become liquid. Place it in a saucepan to liquefy and pour the mixture into the wipes container.
4. Arrange the roll of towels (cut side downward) in a container and add the lid (liquids included).
5. Flip the container for about five minutes for the liquids to penetrate the towels.
6. Open the top of the container to remove the cardboard tube. That part will allow the wipes to pop up as needed.
7. Note: Don't make them too far ahead of time since they could become molded.

#5 Essential Oils & Baby Wipes

Many have found two very effective oils, lavender and chamomile, are safe for your baby. They are also useful in relieving issues such as a diaper rash. You have many options on how to use and store homemade baby wipes and solutions.

Try this nourishing mixture for cleansing your baby's skin:

Materials Needed:
- Distilled or filtered water (1 cup)
- Vitamin E oil as a natural preservative (.25 tsp.)
- Almond/olive/grapeseed oil (1 tbsp.)
- Liquid castile soap (1 tbsp.)
  Essential Oils:
    - Chamomile - Roman (2 drops)
    - Lavender (3 drops)
    - Tea tree oil is another natural preservative (5 drops)

Preparation Steps:
1. Mix each of the fixings, adding water first to avoid creating a batch of bubbles.
2. Use the wipes and solution within one month.
3. Select a technique that works best for you:

    a. Place cloth wipes in a repurposed baby wipe container. Slowly dump the mixture over the wipes until they are moistened, but not drenched. You will probably have an excess of the solution. Save it and add it later if the towels start to dry out.
    b. You can also prepare the solution and add it to a squirt bottle. Shake before use, and squirt directly onto cloth wipes.
    c. The third option is to use a spray bottle. Spray the solution onto cloth wipes before using them

or spray directly onto the child's diaper area,
then wipe with a homemade dry wipe.

#6 Baby Wipes for Two Rolls

Materials Needed:
- Cloth-like paper towels (1 package)
- Boiled water (2 cups)
- Baby bath soap/baby shampoo (1 tbsp.)
- Mineral/baby oil (1 tbsp.)
- Regular/baby lotion (1 tbsp.)
- White vinegar to inhibit mold (1 tbsp.)
- Optional: Tea tree oil (inhibits mold)

Preparation Steps:
1. Use a sharp knife and cut the paper roll in half.
2. Place it in a plastic container with a lid or recycle a baby wipe container.
3. Arrange the shredded side down (to help keep the excess off of the baby's bottom).
4. Pour in the solution.
5. Wait for five minutes and flip the container. The roll of cardboard should be easily removed. Flip the roll back over and pull the center cardboard to start the process.

Other Delightful Oil Fragrances for Baby:

Frankincense essential oil can help with rashes and other skin imperfections.

Rose is a very delicate essential oil for babies' skin.

Wild orange adds a fresh scent and is full of antioxidants; it is also excellent for natural skincare. A word of caution: Don't go outside in the sunlight for a minimum of 12 hours after using the wild orange scent. The same holds with any of the citrus essential oils.

Bonus

Try this alcohol-based scented hand sanitizer lotion:

Materials Needed:
- Rubbing alcohol (10 grams)
- Water (60 grams
- Emulsimulse/any other emulsifying wax (7 grams)
- Glycerin (2 grams)
- Raw honey 3 grams)
- Grapeseed oil (18 grams)
- *Essential Oils Needed*:

    - Tea tree (5 drops)
    - Lavender (8 drops)
    - Rosemary (3 drops)

Preparation Steps:
1. Mix the emulsifying wax and grapeseed oil, and let them melt in a saucepan using the medium temperature setting.
2. Meanwhile, mix the glycerin and water in a microwave-safe bowl. Nuke it for about 20 seconds, stirring it thoroughly to combine.
3. Add and heat the water mixture.
4. Remove the pan from the burner and whisk the mixture constantly as it cools and thickens into a lotion.
5. Whisk in the rubbing alcohol and raw honey. Whisk in the essential oils and pour it into a lotion bottle.

Conclusion

Here we are at the end of our journey through beautiful and fragrant recipes to create your favorite disinfectant. I hope you have enjoyed every chapter and every section of your copy of Hand Sanitizer Recipes.

I intended that this was informative, yes, but above all, easy to read, quick, and easy to put into practice.

I believe you now have all the tools you need to achieve your goals when it comes to preparing an excellent hand sanitizer. But above all, that this allows you to save money compared to having to go to the supermarket or a particular shop to buy them every time secondly, that it is easier for you when you are out and about and do not have toilets, or soap and water available to wash and disinfect.

These operations have become of the utmost necessity in light of the current world health situation brought by the coronavirus.

Personal hygiene, and first and foremost hand washing, can make the difference and sometimes save us from severe consequences.

In the succession of chapters, we have seen the contagion and contact mechanisms, i.e., how germs and viruses can infect us. It has helped us to understand their danger and what we can do to protect our health. We have seen the benefits and comfort of having and using a hand sanitizer, especially when we are out and about and have no soap or water available.

At this point, it was certainly interesting to have understood the types of disinfectants, alcoholic or non-alcoholic, and the differences between them, also in light of what the CDC and WHO recommend in this regard.

We also had the chance to review together the correct technique to wash our hands and disinfect them, taking care to clean all their sensitive spots where viruses and bacteria can lurk most.

So we immersed ourselves in the most creative and fun part, that of recipes to prepare our favorite disinfectants, for fragrance and consistency. With these recipes, you can have fun and maybe start from here to personalize them. We have attached to the recipes useful tips on the user depending on the skin type and for children, whose skin needs special precautions.

You can make your own, undoubtedly, the experience and manual skills in preparing them whenever you need them, but considering the times we live in, I would suggest that you always have one with you when you happen to be out and about. Not to mention the economic savings you make by creating disinfectants at home.

The next step is to put on your following shopping list of basic necessities and start your adventure.

You will also have the motivation to create something useful for you and your loved ones, especially your children, who are the ones who need the most attention concerning hygiene.

I hope you have appreciated the effort in making a recipe book as simple as possible, but full of options and really for all tastes.

Reviews are an author's sap, whatever genre he writes. They allow him to continue writing more helpful books. Without stars and reviews, you would never have found this book. If you would click five stars on your Kindle device, that will ensure that I can continue to produce again, and I sincerely appreciate it.

Please take just twenty seconds of your time to support an independent author by leaving a review on the platform where you purchase this book.

Thank You!

Sincerely,

Paul. S. Leland

As a way of saying thanks for purchasing this book, there is a gift for you: a theme as topical as ever. Discover the dynamics of this sneaky invisible enemy to better protect you and your family.

Simply copy and paste the link below into your browser, to get your gift:

https://dl.bookfunnel.com/spqs3v2rnp

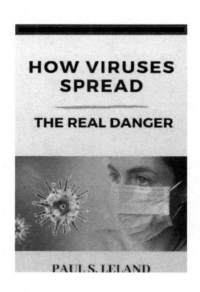

Also available from Paul S. Leland:

- Your Homemade Hand Sanitizer: Quick and Easy, Best Ever Effective Recipes to Protect You and Your Family From Viruses and Bacteria

- Diy Homemade Protective Face Mask: How to Make a True-Effective, Reusable Medical Face Mask with Stuffs You Have at Home

CPSIA information can be obtained
at www.ICGtesting.com
Printed in the USA
BVHW040950121120
593172BV00016B/1765

9 781513 672564